THE CAKE WATCHER

A children's story about gestational surrogacy
and growing your family

BY JESSICA ROSENBERG

They say it takes a village
and for us that was certainly true.
So when I look at our beautiful boys
I am eternally grateful for all of you.

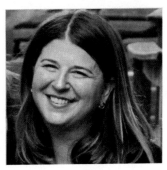

Jessica Rosenberg

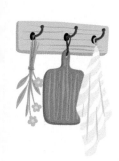

Leo, Mommy, and Papa
were buzzing around the kitchen.
They were on a mission
to bake a cake with more precision.

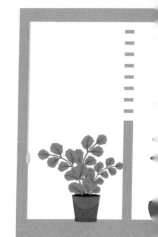

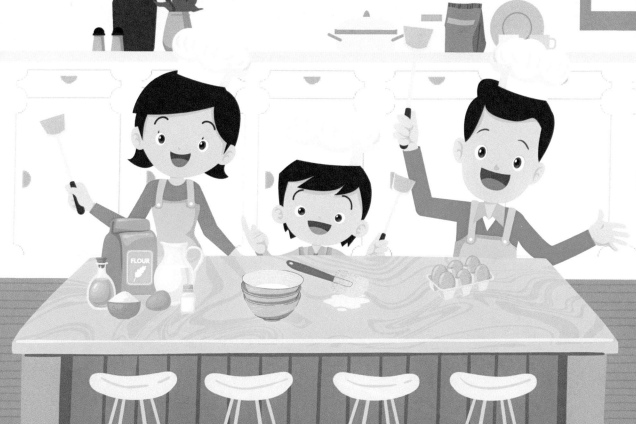

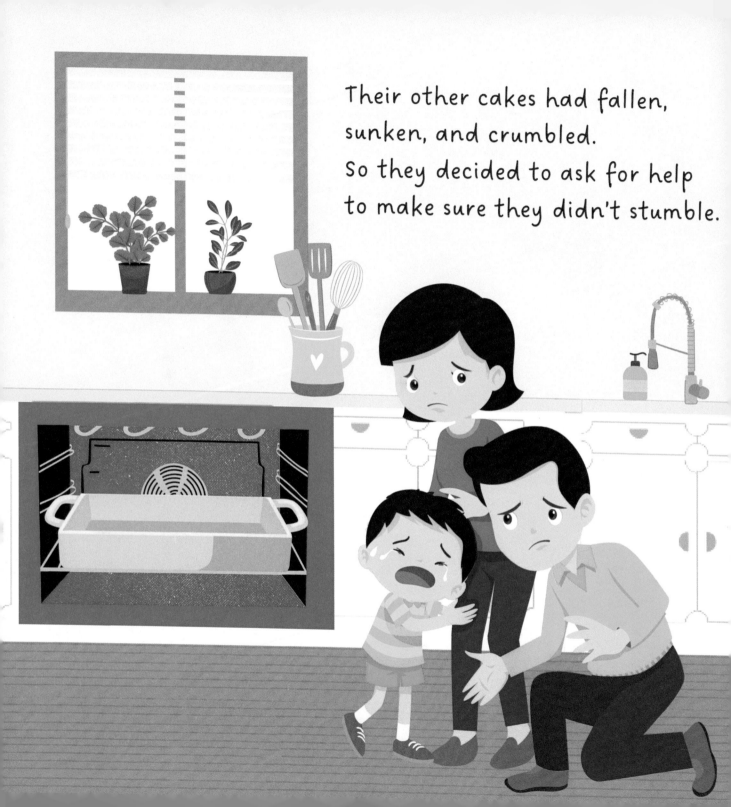

Their other cakes had fallen,
sunken, and crumbled.
So they decided to ask for help
to make sure they didn't stumble.

First, they called Chef Lia
to help them with their recipe.

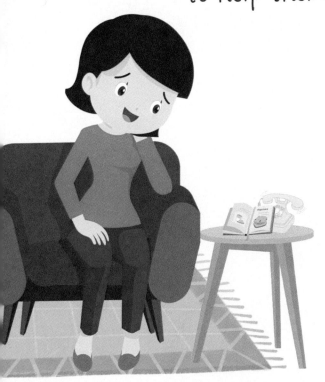
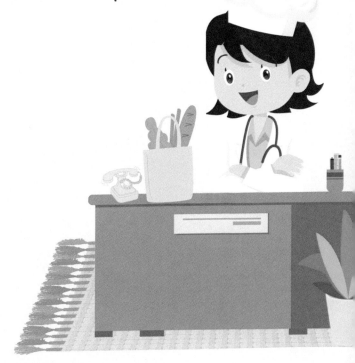

They gathered the ingredients
and measured everything steadily.

They mixed, stirred, whisked, and
mixed it up some more...
Filling the kitchen with laughter,
and dreams of being a family of four.

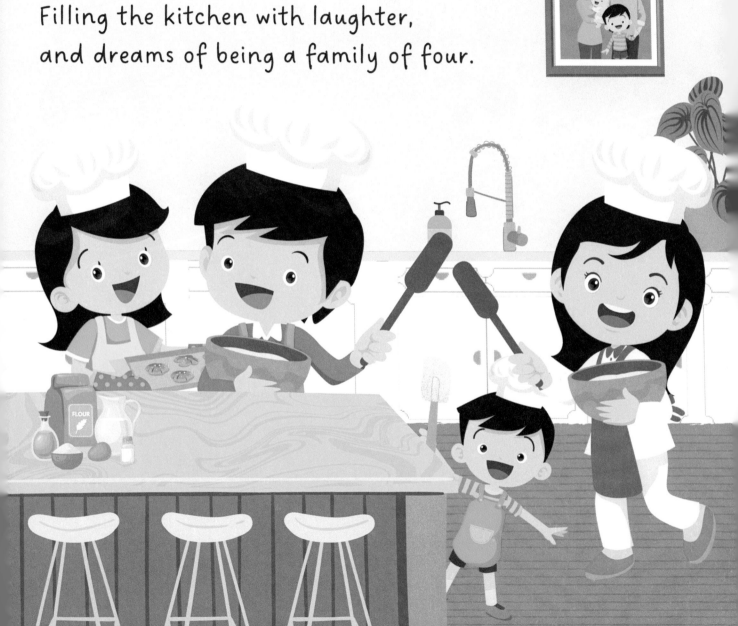

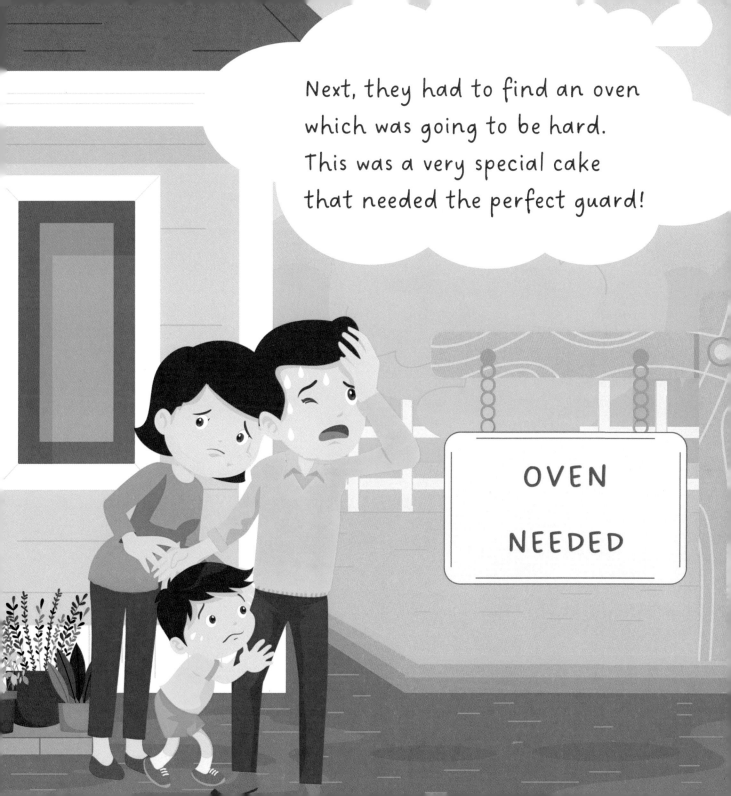

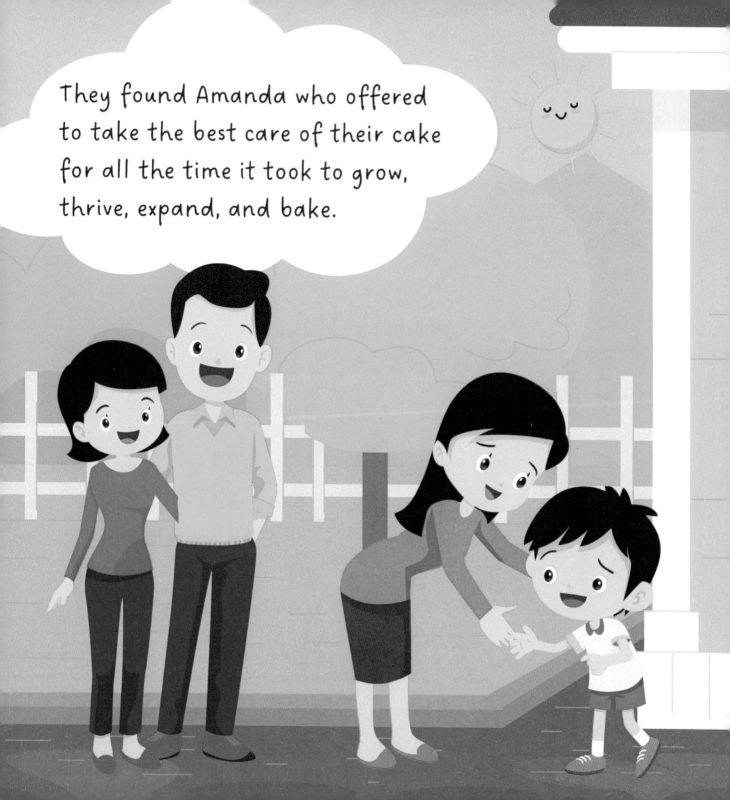

They found Amanda who offered to take the best care of their cake for all the time it took to grow, thrive, expand, and bake.

They brought their cake pan over
with excitement and fanfare.
Amanda gently placed it in her oven
and set the temperature with care.

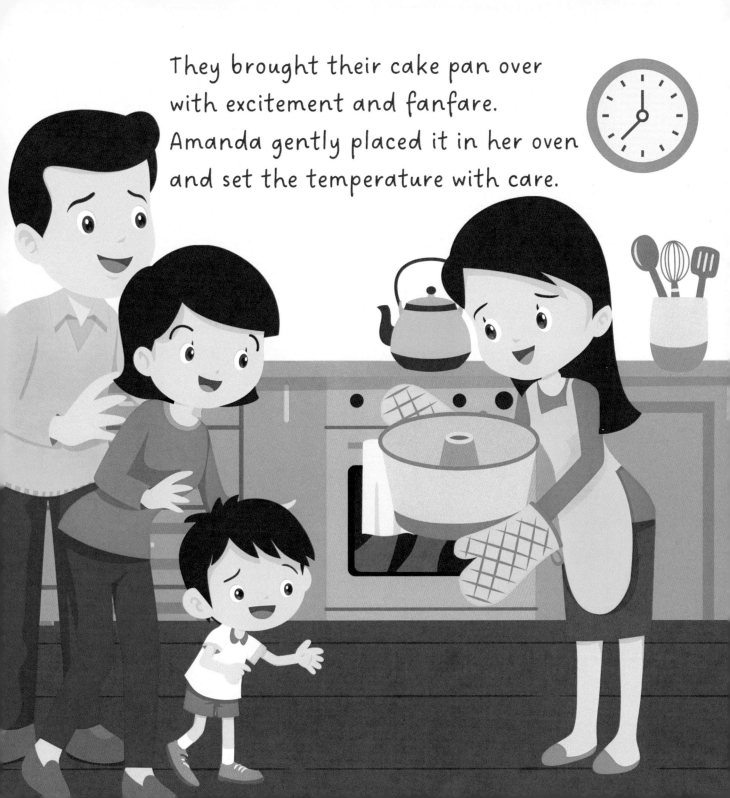

Now that their cake was baking,
they were relieved and felt great.
So with a big hug for Amanda,
the family went home to wait.

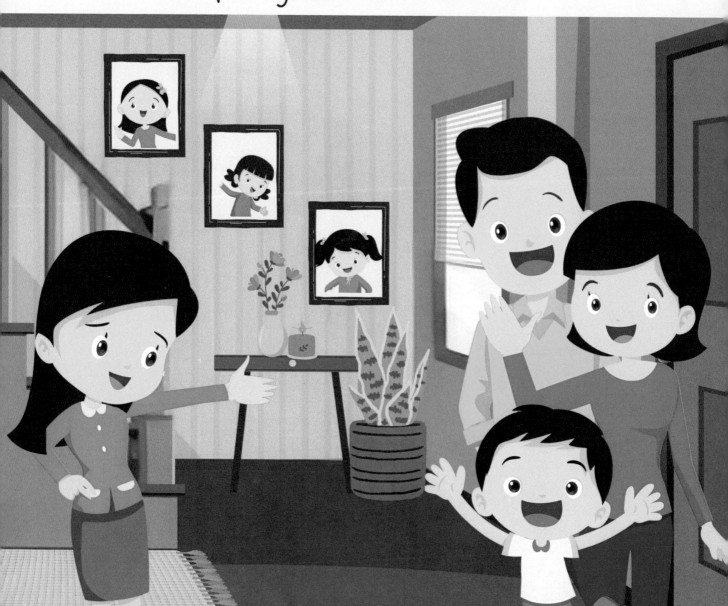

Amanda closely watched her oven,
eyes sparkling with responsibility.
She turned the cake when needed
and checked the temperature consistently.

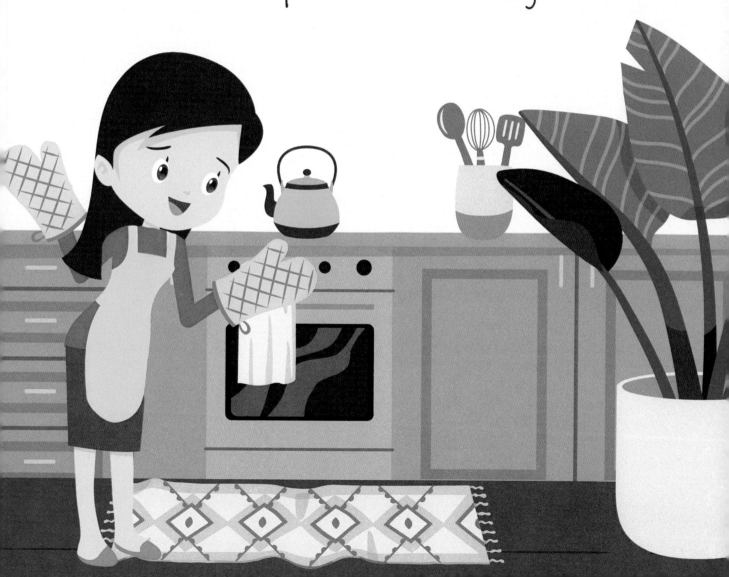

She gave it words of encouragement
and kept the family updated
with frequent messages and pictures,
knowing how patiently they've waited.

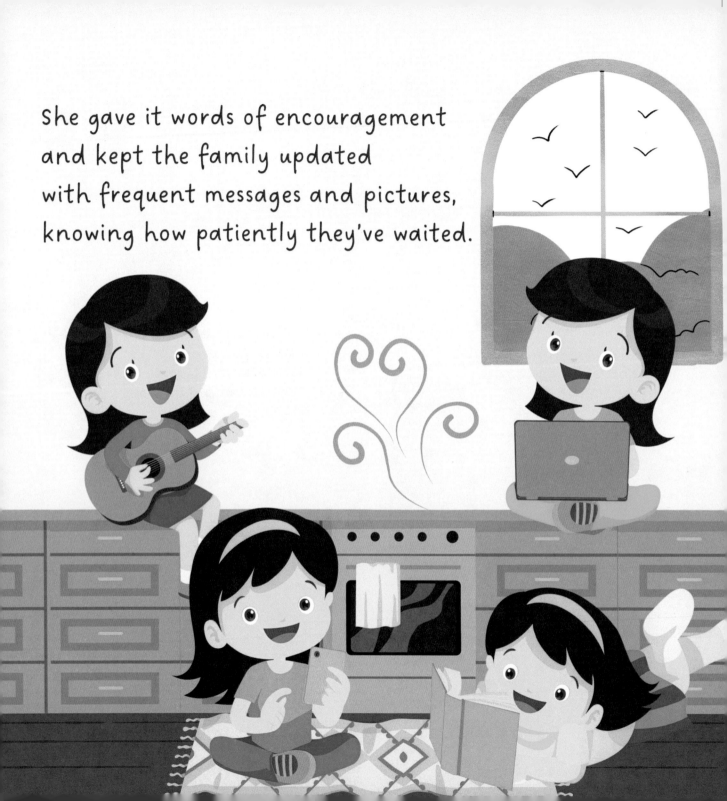

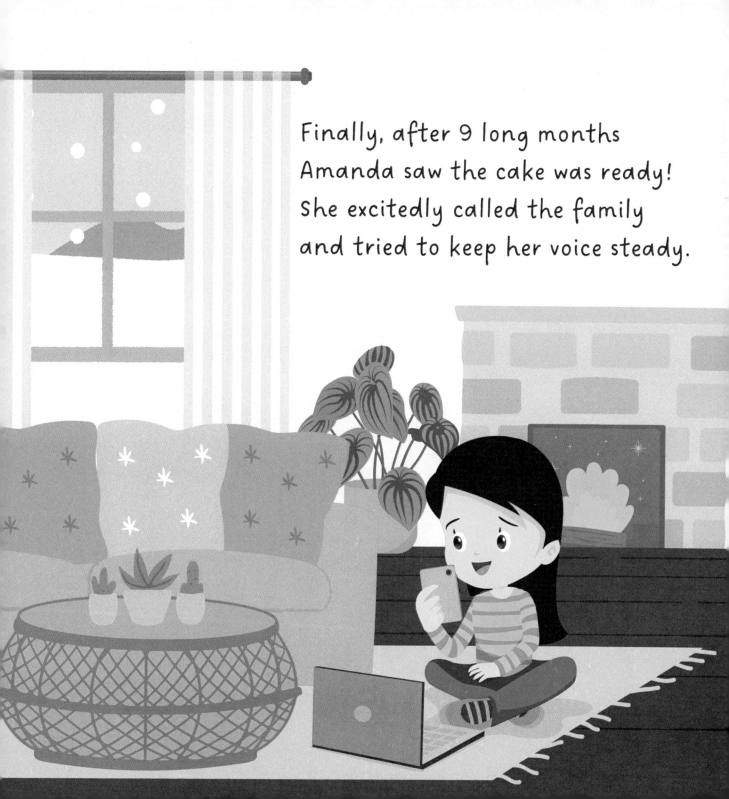

Finally, after 9 long months
Amanda saw the cake was ready!
She excitedly called the family
and tried to keep her voice steady.

As she shared the exciting news,
the family was overcome with emotion.
They rushed over, their eyes twinkling,
so grateful for Amanda's devotion.

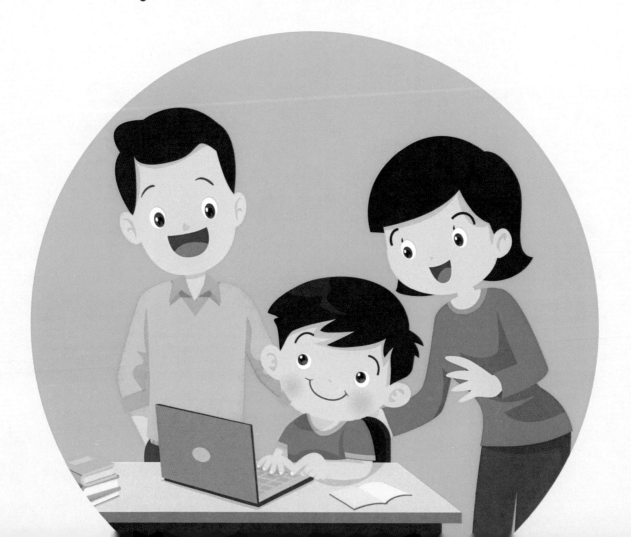

As they all worked together
to remove the cake hand in hand
they admired the beautiful cake
which was even better than they planned.

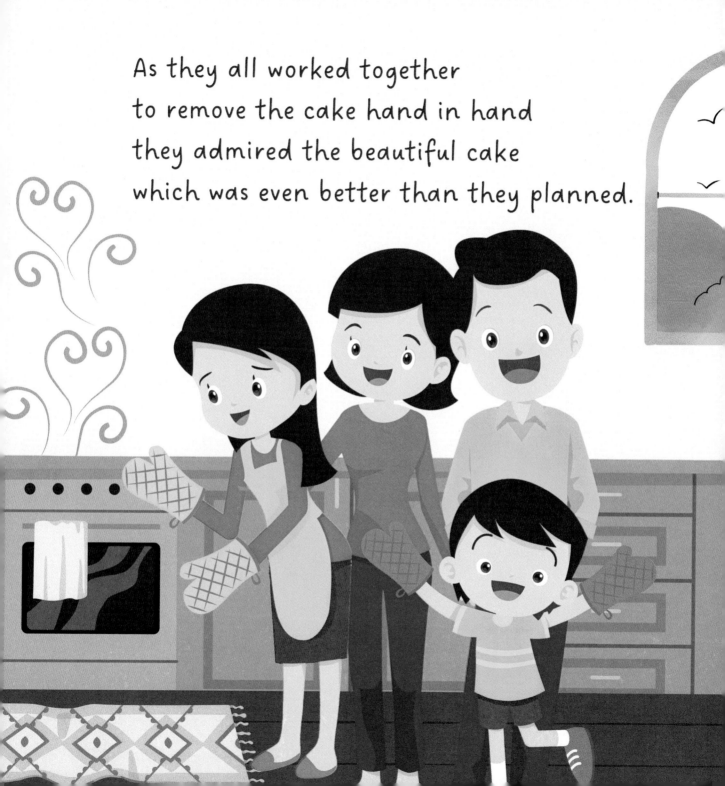

And when they set down the finished cake
their faces lit up with joy.
It was perfect! A rainbow cake
to welcome a special baby boy.

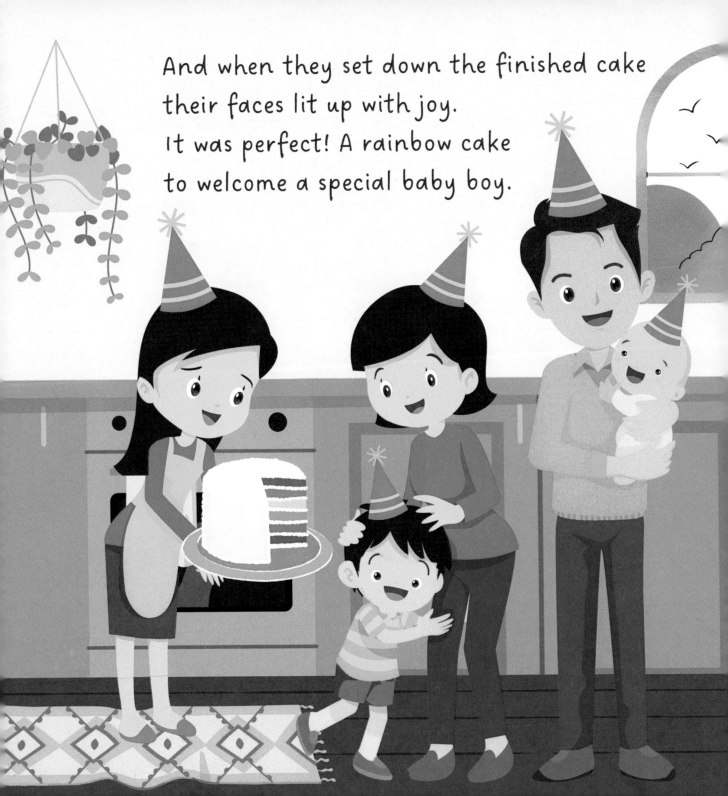

As they left they hugged Amanda
for she gave them such a gift.
Amanda was sad to see them go
but seeing their joy made her feelings shift.

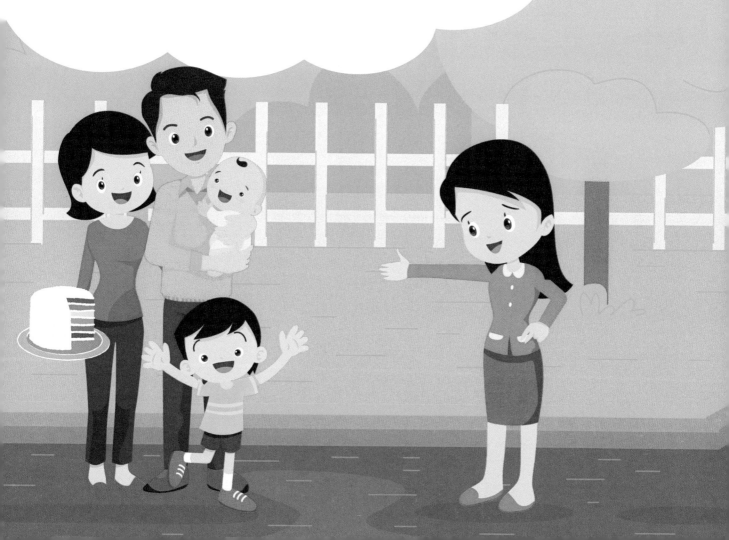

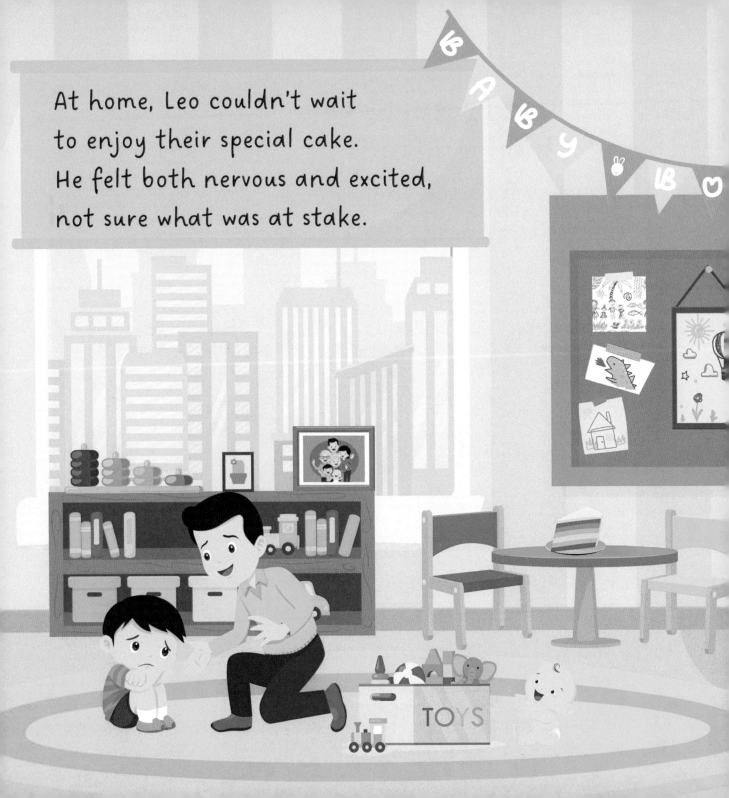

At home, Leo couldn't wait
to enjoy their special cake.
He felt both nervous and excited,
not sure what was at stake.

But when he looked up at his parents
and saw their loving smiles,
he knew their family would grow together
no matter what the trials.

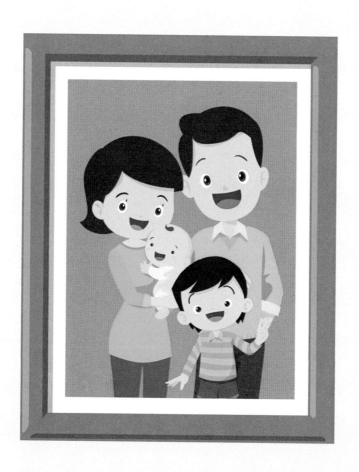

Made in the USA
Las Vegas, NV
09 December 2024

13734397R00017